THE KIDNE

MW00876256

DIET COOKBOOK

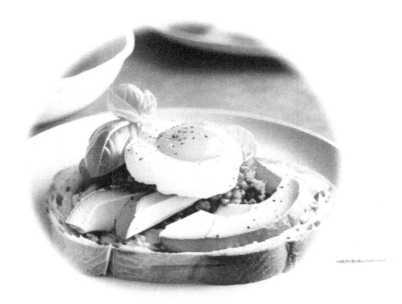

**Meal Plans with Complete Nutrition
Guide Recipes for Transplant
Patients, to Manage and Improve
Renal Functions and to Prevent
Complications**

Dr. Pamela Elliott

Copyright © 2023 by Dr. Pamela Elliott

All Rights Reserved

This literary work is protected by copyright laws and is provided solely for the private use of the original owner.

Unauthorized copying, adaptation, distribution, public performance, or other use of this work is strictly prohibited and may result in civil and/or criminal penalties.

Table of Contents

Introduction **10**

CHAPTER ONE **17**

Kidney Transplant Diet 17

Benefits of a Kidney Transplant Diet.... 19

General Guidelines for a Kidney Transplant Diet................................ 21

Tips to Kidney Transplant Diets 24

CHAPTER TWO **30**

7-Days Kidney Transplant Diet Meal Plan **30**

Day 1 ....**30**

Breakfast: Spinach and Feta Omelet ... 30

Lunch: Roasted Vegetable and Quinoa Salad 32

Dinner: Grilled Salmon with Lemon Dill Sauce 33

Day 2 ....**35**

Breakfast: Avocado Toast with Poached Egg 35

Lunch: Lentil Soup 36

Dinner: Baked Cod with Tomato and Herb Sauce 38

Day 3 ....**40**

Breakfast: Berry Smoothie 40

Lunch: Quinoa and Black Bean Salad... 41

Dinner: Grilled Vegetables and Rice 43

Day 4 ....**45**

Breakfast: Overnight Oats................. 45

Lunch: Broccoli and Cheddar Frittata... 47

Dinner: Zucchini Noodles with Pesto.... 48

Day 5 ....**50**

Breakfast: Greek Yogurt Parfait 50

Lunch: Chickpea and Spinach Salad 51

Dinner: Baked Fish with Lemon and Thyme... 53

Day 6 ....**55**

Breakfast: Oatmeal with Berries 55

Lunch: Lentil and Vegetable Soup 57

Dinner: Baked Tofu and Vegetables..... 58

Day 7 ....**60**

Breakfast: Smoothie Bowl.................. 60

Lunch: Veggie Wrap.......................... 61

Dinner: Roasted Salmon with Lemon and Dill.. 63

CHAPTER THREE **65**

Breakfast Recipes for Kidney Transplant Diets 65

1. 40-Second Omelet: 65

2. Anytime Energy Bars: 66

3. Apple Bran Muffins: 68

4. Banana-Apple Smoothie: 70

5. Banana Oat Shake: 71

6. Berrylicious Smoothie: 72

7. Blueberry Oatmeal: 73

8. Burritos Rapidos: 75

9. Fresh Fruit Lassi: 77

10. Apple Filled Crepes: 78

CHAPTER FOUR **80**

Lunch Recipes for Kidney Transplant Diets 80

1. Apple Rice Salad 80

2. Baked Potato Soup 82

3. Beef Barley Soup 84

4. Black Bean Burger 86

5. Chicken and Corn Chowder 88

6. Chicken and Dumplings 90

7. Chicken N' Orange Salad Sandwich . 92

8. Chinese Chicken Salad 94

9. Cider Cream Chicken 96

10. Dijon Chicken Salad 98

CHAPTER FIVE **100**

Dinner Recipes for Kidney Transplant Diets 100

1. Confetti Chicken 'N Rice 100

2. Crock Pot Chili Verde 102

3. Dilled Fish 104

4.   Easy Instant Pot Creamy Chicken Pasta 106

5.   Fast Fajitas........................ 108

6. Fast Roast Chicken with Lemon & Herbs............................ 111

7. Fresh Marinara Sauce 112

8. Fruit Vinegar Chicken 114

9. Fruity Chicken Salad................... 116

10. Grilled Salmon with Fruit Salsa ... 118

CHAPTER Six........................**120**

Desserts Recipes for Kidney Transplant Diets 120

1. Asian Pear Torte 120

2. Blueberry Whipped Pie................ 122

3. Caramel Custard 124

4. Carrot Muffins........................... 126

5.   Cheesecake 128

CHAPTER Seven **131**

Snacks Recipes for Kidney Transplant Diets 131

1. Beef Jerky 131

2. Brown Bag Popcorn 133

3. Cornbread Muffins....................... 134

4. Ginger Cranberry Punch............... 136

5. Joyce's Quick Dip 138

Conclusion **140**

Introduction

John was a healthy and active young man who had just turned 30.

He was living a normal life until he was diagnosed with kidney failure. His doctor informed him that he would need to receive a kidney transplant in order to survive.

John was devastated by the news, but he was determined to do whatever it took to get the transplant.

He started researching different diets that might help him prepare for the transplant and after.

He found one that seemed promising. He began following the diet and was soon able to get on the waiting list for a kidney transplant.

Months passed and John's health was slowly deteriorating, but he kept up with the diet and waited patiently for a donor.

Finally, after months of waiting, a donor was found and the transplant was a success.

John was amazed at how quickly his body responded to the new kidney and how quickly he was able to recover.

John continues to eat from the kidney transplant diet.

He continues with the diet to keep receiving the necessary nutrients for proper functioning.

The diet also helps to minimize the risk of developing complications from the transplant.

John was even more amazed at how well he was able to manage his diet to ensure that he was getting the nutrients he needed to stay healthy.

John was so thankful for the successful transplant and for the diet that helped him stay healthy.

He was also thankful for the donor who gave him a second chance at life. He was now able to live life to the fullest and enjoy every moment.

John was now an example to others in his situation.

He had managed to beat the odds and successfully manage a kidney transplant with the right diet. He was an inspiration to all.

Welcome to the Kidney Transplant Diet Cookbook!

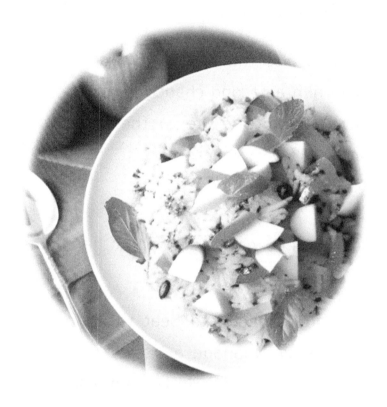

In this book, you will find delicious and nutritious recipes to help you adjust to your new kidney-friendly diet.

As a kidney transplant patient, it's important to understand the importance of eating a well-balanced and nutritious diet.

Not only does a healthy diet help ensure that your body is receiving the necessary nutrients for proper function, but it also helps to minimize the risk of developing complications from your transplant.

This cookbook is designed to give you the tools to create meals that are both tasty and beneficial for your new diet.

You'll find a variety of recipes designed to meet the specific dietary needs of kidney transplant patients, including those that are low in sodium, potassium, and phosphorus.

You'll also learn about proper portion control, hydration, and ways to eat nutritiously while still enjoying the foods you love.

Most importantly, you'll gain the confidence to prepare meals that are both delicious and tailored to your specific dietary needs.

So, let's get cooking! We hope you enjoy the recipes in this cookbook and find them beneficial to your new lifestyle.

CHAPTER ONE

Kidney Transplant Diet

A kidney transplant is a surgical procedure that involves the removal of a healthy kidney from a donor and its placement into a recipient whose own kidneys are no longer functioning adequately.

A successful kidney transplant can restore normal kidney function and improve quality of life for the recipient.

It can also save the recipient from having to go through dialysis treatments.

After a kidney transplant, it is important for the recipient to follow a diet that is tailored to their needs.

This diet should be designed to provide the necessary nutrition while also managing any potential side effects or complications.

It should also be supplemented with a regular exercise program.

The following article will provide an overview of the general dietary guidelines for a successful kidney transplant.

Benefits of a Kidney Transplant Diet

A kidney transplant diet should be designed to provide the necessary nutrients to keep the recipient healthy and to prevent any potential complications.

This diet should focus on limiting sodium and protein intake, as well as avoiding foods that may be high in potassium.

Additionally, the diet should be tailored to meet the individual needs of the recipient, such as ensuring adequate hydration levels and providing sufficient calories to maintain a healthy weight.

A kidney transplant diet should also focus on providing the necessary vitamins and minerals for the body to heal and function properly.

The diet should include foods that are high in vitamins A, B, and C, as well as minerals such as zinc, magnesium, and iron.

Additionally, the diet should include foods that are high in antioxidants, such as fruits and vegetables, to help protect against any infections or other complications.

General Guidelines for a Kidney Transplant Diet

The general guidelines for a kidney transplant diet should include the following:

1. A diet with adequate hydration: Adequate hydration is essential for a successful kidney transplant. The recipient should aim to drink 8-10 glasses of water per day and should avoid drinking too much alcohol or caffeine.

2. A diet low in sodium and protein: Eating a diet that is low in sodium and protein can help to reduce the risk of complications and can promote better kidney function. It is important to limit processed foods and to choose foods that are naturally low in sodium and protein.

3. A diet that is rich in vitamins and minerals: Eating a diet that is rich in vitamins and minerals can help to promote better kidney function and can help to prevent any potential complications. Foods that are high in vitamins and minerals include fruits and vegetables, whole grains, lean proteins, nuts, and seeds.

4. A diet that is low in potassium: Eating a diet that is low in potassium can help to reduce the risk of any potential complications. Foods that are high in potassium should be avoided, such as bananas, potatoes, tomatoes, and orange juice.

5. A diet that is supplemented with regular exercise: Regular exercise can help to promote better kidney function and can help to reduce the risk of any potential complications. Exercise should be done regularly and should include both aerobic and strength training activities.

Tips to Kidney Transplant Diets

A kidney transplant diet is a specialized meal plan that is tailored to meet the specific needs of someone who was about to get the kidney tansplant or who recently undergone a kidney transplant.

It is important to follow a kidney transplant diet to ensure that the body is getting the proper nutrition it needs to heal and recover from the surgery and to prevent any complications.

The following are some tips for following a kidney transplant diet:

- **Consume adequate amounts of protein:** Protein is essential for healing and maintaining healthy tissue after a transplant. Aim to consume between 0.8 and 1.2 grams of protein per kilogram of body weight per day, depending on the individual's needs.

- **Get enough calcium and vitamin D:** Getting adequate calcium and vitamin D is important for bone health, especially after a transplant. Aim to get at least 1,000 milligrams of calcium per day and 400 to 800 international units of vitamin D. Sources of calcium and vitamin D include fortified milk, yogurt, cheese, and fortified breakfast cereals.

- **Consume healthy fats:** Healthy fats, such as olive oil, canola oil, nuts, seeds, and fish, can help to provide essential fatty acids that the body needs. Aim to get at least 20 to 35 percent of daily calories from healthy fats.

- **Avoid processed foods:** Processed foods are usually high in sodium and not a good source of nutrients, so it's best to avoid them.

- **Monitor your sodium intake:** High-sodium foods can increase blood pressure, so it's important to monitor your sodium intake. Consume not more than 2,000 milligrams of sodium per day.

- **Eat plenty of fruits and vegetables:** Fruits and vegetables are a great source of vitamins, minerals, and fiber. Consume at least five servings of fruits and vegetables per day.

- **Drink plenty of fluids:** It's important to drink plenty of fluids to help keep your body hydrated and to help with kidney function. Drink at least eight glasses of water per day.

- **Avoid alcohol:** It's best to avoid alcohol completely after a kidney transplant.

- **Avoid caffeine:** Caffeine can cause dehydration and can increase blood pressure, so it's best to avoid it.

- **Take your medications as directed:** It's important to take your medications as directed by your doctor to help prevent any complications or rejection of the transplant.

- **Keep a food journal:** Keeping a food journal can help you to monitor your food intake and can help you to make sure that you're getting the proper nutrition.

- **Talk to your doctor: If you have any** questions or concerns about your diet, it's important to talk to your doctor. They can provide you with more specific advice and can help to ensure that you're getting the proper nutrition.

CHAPTER TWO

7-Days Kidney Transplant Diet Meal Plan

Day 1

Breakfast: Spinach and Feta Omelet

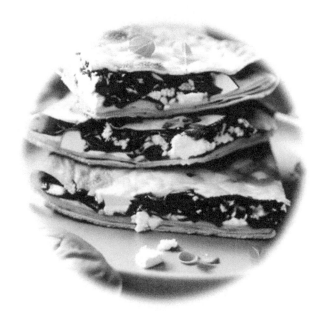

Ingredients:

- 2 eggs,

- 1/4 cup crumbled feta cheese,

- 1/4 cup chopped spinach,

- 2 tablespoons olive oil,

- Salt and pepper to taste

Preparation:

- Heat the olive oil in a skillet on average heat.

- Add the spinach and cook until wilted.

- Beat the eggs together in a bowl with feta cheese, salt and pepper.

- Pour the egg mixture into the skillet and cook until firm, flipping once.

Lunch: Roasted Vegetable and Quinoa Salad

Ingredients:

- 1 cup cooked quinoa,

- 1/2 cup diced carrots,

- 1/2 cup diced bell peppers,

- 1/2 cup diced zucchini,

- 1/4 cup diced onion,

- 2 tablespoons olive oil,

- Salt and pepper to taste

Preparation:

- Preheat oven to 375F.

- Toss the carrots, bell peppers, zucchini, and onion with olive oil, salt and pepper.

- Spread onto a baking sheet and roast for 15 minutes.

- In a bowl, combine the roasted vegetables with the cooked quinoa.

- Serve warm or chilled.

Dinner: Grilled Salmon with Lemon Dill Sauce

Ingredients:

- 2 salmon filets,

- 2 tablespoons olive oil,

- 1/4 cup fresh lemon juice,

- 1 tablespoon minced fresh dill,

- Salt and pepper to taste

Preparation:

- Heat the olive oil in a skillet over medium heat.

- Season the salmon with salt and pepper and cook for 8-10 minutes, flipping once.

- Meanwhile, mix the lemon juice, dill, salt and pepper in a small bowl.

- Pour the sauce over the salmon and cook for an additional 2 minutes.

- Serve hot.

Day 2

Breakfast: Avocado Toast with Poached Egg

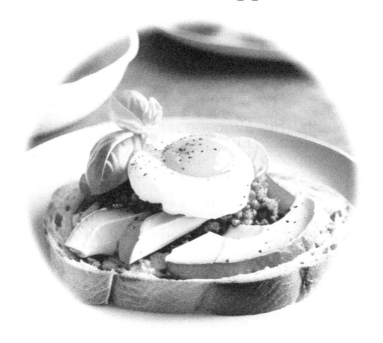

Ingredients:

- 2 slices whole-grain bread,

- 1 avocado,

- 1 teaspoon olive oil,

- 1 poached egg,

- Salt and pepper to taste

Preparation:

- Toast the bread slices.

- Mash the avocado with olive oil, salt and pepper and spread on top of the toasted bread.

- Top with a poached egg and serve.

Lunch: Lentil Soup

Ingredients:

- 1 tablespoon olive oil,

- 1/2 cup diced onion,

- 1 cup diced carrots,

- 1 cup diced celery,

- 1/2 cup red lentils,

- 4 cups vegetable broth,

- 1/2 teaspoon dried thyme,

- Salt and pepper to taste

Preparation:

- Heat the olive oil in a large pot over medium heat.

- Add the onion, carrots, and celery and cook for 5 minutes.

- Add the lentils, broth, and thyme. Bring to a boil, reduce heat and simmer for 25 minutes.

- Season with salt and pepper to taste. Serve warm.

Dinner: Baked Cod with Tomato and Herb Sauce

Ingredients:

- 2 cod filets,

- 2 tablespoons olive oil,

- 1/4 cup diced tomatoes,

- 2 tablespoons minced fresh herbs (parsley, basil, oregano),

- Salt and pepper to taste

Preparation:

• Preheat oven to 375F.

• Place the cod filets in a baking dish. Drizzle with olive oil and season with salt and pepper.

• In a small bowl, mix together the tomatoes, herbs, salt and pepper.

• Spread the tomato mixture over the cod.

• Bake for 15 minutes, or until the fish is cooked through.

• Serve hot.

Day 3

Breakfast: Berry Smoothie

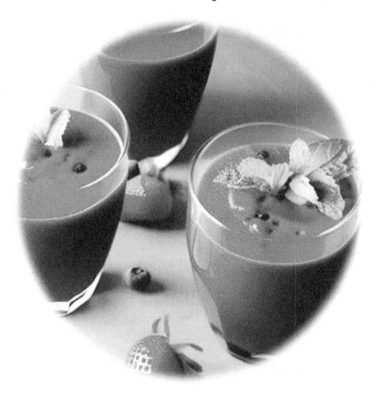

Ingredients:

- 1 cup frozen berries,

- 1/2 cup plain Greek yogurt,

- 1/2 cup almond milk,

- 1 tablespoon honey

Preparation:

- Place all ingredients in a blender

- Blend until smooth. Serve cold.

Lunch: Quinoa and Black Bean Salad

Ingredients:

- 1 cup cooked quinoa,

- 1/2 cup cooked black beans,

- 1/4 cup diced red bell pepper,

- 1/4 cup diced red onion,

- 2 tablespoons olive oil,

- 2 tablespoons freshly squeezed lime juice,

- 1 tablespoon minced cilantro,

- Salt and pepper to taste

Preparation:

- In a large bowl, combine the quinoa, black beans, bell pepper, and onion.

- In a bowl, whisk together the olive oil, the lime juice, the cilantro, salt and pepper.

- Pour the dressing on the salad and toss it to combine.

- Serve cold or at room temperature.

Dinner: Grilled Vegetables and Rice

Ingredients:

- 2 cups cooked brown rice,

- 1/2 cup diced carrots,

- 1/2 cup diced bell peppers,

- 1/2 cup diced zucchini,

- 1/4 cup diced onion,

- 2 tablespoons olive oil,

- Salt and pepper to taste

Preparation:

• Heat a grill or grill pan to medium-high heat.

• Toss the carrots, bell peppers, zucchini, and onion with olive oil, salt and pepper.

• Grill the vegetables for 10 minutes, or until tender, flipping once.

• Serve the grilled vegetables over the cooked brown rice.

Day 4

Breakfast: Overnight Oats

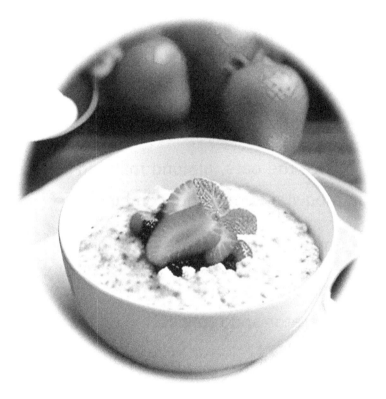

Ingredients:

- 1/2 cup rolled oats,

- 1/2 cup almond milk,

- 1 tablespoon honey,

- 1/4 cup mixed berries

Preparation:

- Place the oats, almond milk, and honey in a bowl and mix until combined.

- Cover and refrigerate overnight.

- In the morning, remove from the refrigerator and top with mixed berries.

- Serve chilled.

Lunch: Broccoli and Cheddar Frittata

Ingredients:

- 2 eggs,

- 1/2 cup cooked broccoli,

- 1/4 cup shredded cheddar cheese,

- 2 tablespoons olive oil,

- Salt and pepper to taste

Preparation:

- Heat the olive oil in a skillet on average heat.

- Beat the eggs together in a bowl with the cheese, salt and pepper.

- Pour the egg mixture into the skillet and top with the cooked broccoli.

- Cook until firm, flipping once.

- Serve hot.

Dinner: Zucchini Noodles with Pesto

Ingredients:

- 2 medium zucchinis,

- 2 tablespoons olive oil,

- 1/4 cup prepared pesto,

- Salt and pepper to taste

Preparation:

• Using a spiralizer or mandoline, cut the zucchinis into noodles.

• Heat the olive oil in a skillet on average heat.

• Add the zucchini noodles and cook for 5 minutes, or until tender.

• Toss with the pesto and season with salt and pepper to taste.

• Serve hot.

Day 5

Breakfast: Greek Yogurt Parfait

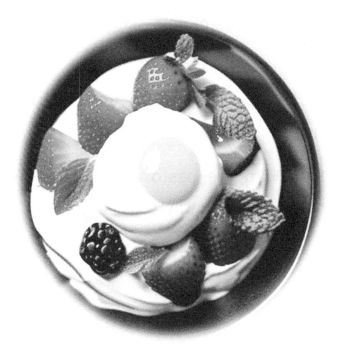

Ingredients:

- 1/2 cup plain Greek yogurt,

- 1/4 cup granola,

- 1/4 cup mixed berries

Preparation:

- Layer the Greek yogurt, granola, and berries in a bowl.

- Serve chilled.

Lunch: Chickpea and Spinach Salad

Ingredients:

- 1 can of chickpeas,

- 1/2 cup chopped spinach,

- 1/4 cup diced red onion,

- 2 tablespoons olive oil,

- 2 tablespoons freshly squeezed lemon juice,

- 1 teaspoon minced garlic,

- Salt and pepper to taste

Preparation:

- Drain and rinse the chickpeas.

- In a large bowl, combine the chickpeas, spinach, and onion.

- In a bowl, whisk together the olive oil, the lemon juice, the garlic, salt and pepper.

- Pour the dressing on the salad and toss it to combine.

- Serve cold or at room temperature.

Dinner: Baked Fish with Lemon and Thyme

Ingredients:

- 2 white fish filets,

- 2 tablespoons olive oil,

- 1/4 cup freshly squeezed lemon juice,

- 1 tablespoon minced fresh thyme,

- Salt and pepper to taste

Preparation:

- Preheat oven to 375F.

- Place fish filets in a baking dish.

- Drizzle it with olive oil and season it with salt and with pepper.

- In a small bowl, mix together the lemon juice, thyme, salt and pepper.

- Pour the sauce over the fish.

- Bake it for 15 minutes, or till the fish is cooked through.

- Serve hot.

Day 6

Breakfast: Oatmeal with Berries

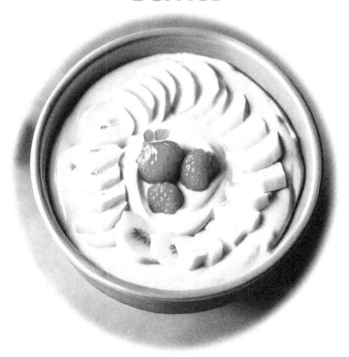

Ingredients:

- 1/2 cup rolled oats,

- 1 cup almond milk,

- 1 tablespoon honey,

- 1/4 cup mixed berries

Preparation:

- Place the oats and almond milk in a saucepan and bring to a boil.

- Reduce heat and simmer for 5 minutes. Remove it from heat and then stir in the honey.

- Serve warm, topped with mixed berries.

Lunch: Lentil and Vegetable Soup

Ingredients:

- 1 tablespoon olive oil,

- 1/2 cup diced onion,

- 1 cup diced carrots,

- 1 cup diced celery,

- 1/2 cup red lentils,

- 4 cups vegetable broth,

- 1/2 teaspoon dried thyme,

- Salt and pepper to taste

- **Preparation:**

Heat the olive oil in a bigger pot on average heat.

- Add the onion, the carrots, and the celery and cook it for 5 minutes.

- Add the lentils, broth, and thyme. Bring to boil and then reduce the heat and simmer it for like 25 minutes.

- Season it with salt and with pepper to taste. Serve warm.

Dinner: Baked Tofu and Vegetables

Ingredients:

- 1 package extra-firm tofu,

- 1/2 cup diced carrots,

- 1/2 cup diced bell peppers,

- 1/2 cup diced zucchini,

- 1/4 cup diced onion,

- 2 tablespoons olive oil,

- Salt and pepper to taste

- Preparation:

- Preheat oven to 375F.

- Drain the tofu and cut into cubes.

- Toss the carrots, bell peppers, zucchini, and onion with olive oil, salt and pepper.

- Spread on a baking sheet and bake it for like 15 minutes.

- Add the tofu to the baking sheet and bake for an additional 10 minutes. Serve hot.

Day 7

Breakfast: Smoothie Bowl

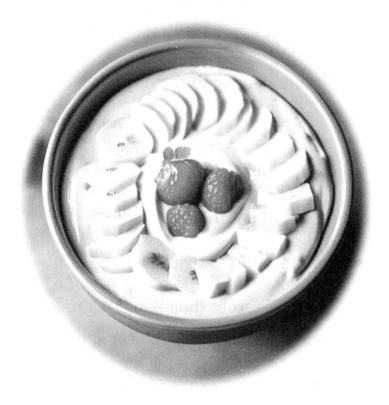

Ingredients:

- 1 banana,

- 1/2 cup plain Greek yogurt,

- 1/2 cup almond milk,

- 1 tablespoon honey,

- 1/4 cup mixed berries

Preparation:

- Place all ingredients in a blender

- Blend until smooth.

- Serve in a bowl with additional mixed berries.

Lunch: Veggie Wrap

Ingredients:

- 2 whole-wheat tortillas,

- 1/2 cup diced tomatoes,

- 1/2 cup diced cucumber,

- 1/4 cup diced red onion,

- 2 tablespoons freshly squeezed lemon juice,

- 1 tablespoon minced fresh herbs (parsley, basil, oregano),

- Salt and pepper to taste

Preparation:

- In a bowl, combine the tomatoes, cucumber, and onion.

- In a small bowl, whisk together the lemon juice, herbs, salt and pepper.

- Pour the dressing over the vegetables and toss to combine.

- Place the vegetables on the tortillas and wrap. Serve cold or at room temperature.

Dinner: Roasted Salmon with Lemon and Dill

Ingredients:

- 2 salmon filets,

- 2 tablespoons olive oil,

- 1/4 cup freshly squeezed lemon juice,

- 1 tablespoon minced fresh dill,

- Salt and pepper to taste

Preparation:

- Preheat oven to 375F. Place salmon filets in a baking dish.

- Drizzle with olive oil and season with salt and pepper.

- In a small bowl, mix together the lemon juice, dill, salt and pepper.

- Pour the sauce over the salmon and bake for 15 minutes, or until the fish is cooked through.

- Serve hot.

CHAPTER THREE

Breakfast Recipes for Kidney Transplant Diets

1. 40-Second Omelet:

Ingredients:

- 2 eggs

- 2 tablespoons milk

- 2 tablespoons chopped vegetables (such as bell pepper, onion, mushrooms, etc.)

- 2 tablespoons shredded cheese (optional)

- Salt and pepper to taste

Preparation:

- In a microwavable mug, whisk together the eggs, milk, vegetables, and cheese (if using).

- Season with salt and pepper. Microwave on high for 40 seconds, stirring after 20 seconds.

- Serve immediately.

2. Anytime Energy Bars:

Ingredients:

- 2 cups rolled oats

- 1/2 cup nut butter

- 1/2 cup honey

- 1/2 cup chopped nuts (such as almonds, walnuts, etc.)

- 1/2 cup dried fruit (such as raisins, cranberries, etc.)

- 1/2 cup chocolate chips (optional)

Preparation:

- In a medium bowl, mix together the rolled oats, nut butter, honey, nuts, and dried fruit.

- Stir in the chocolate chips (if using). Grease an 8x8-inch of baking dish with the oil spray.

- Press the mixture into the dish.

- Refrigerate it for at least 1 hour before cutting it into bars.

3. Apple Bran Muffins:

Ingredients:

- 2 cups all-purpose flour

- 1 cup wheat bran

- 1 teaspoon baking soda

- 1 teaspoon baking powder

- 1/4 teaspoon salt

- 1/2 cup melted butter

- 1/2 cup brown sugar

- 2 eggs

- 1 cup buttermilk

- 1 cup diced apples

Preparation:

• Preheat oven to 375°F. Grease a 12-cup muffin tin.

• In a bigger bowl, whisk together the flour, the wheat bran, the baking soda, the baking powder, and salt.

• In a separate bowl, whisk together the melted butter and brown sugar.

Add the eggs and buttermilk, and whisk until combined.

• Add the wet ingredients to with the dry ingredients, and the mix till just combined.

• Fold in the diced apples. Fill each muffin cup with the batter.

- Bake it for like 18-20 minutes, or till a toothpick inserted into the center can comes out clean.

- Allow to cool before serving.

4. Banana-Apple Smoothie:

Ingredients:

- 1 banana

- 1 apple, peeled and diced

- 1 cup plain yogurt

- 1/2 cup orange juice

- 2 tablespoons honey

Preparation:

- In a blender, combine the banana, apple, yogurt, orange juice, and honey.

- Blend until smooth. Serve immediately.

5. Banana Oat Shake:

Ingredients:

- 1 banana

- 1/2 cup rolled oats

- 1 cup milk

- 1 teaspoon honey

- 1/2 teaspoon vanilla extract

Preparation:

- In a blender, combine the banana, oats, milk, honey, and vanilla extract.

- Blend until smooth. Serve immediately.

6. Berrylicious Smoothie:

Ingredients:

- 1 cup mixed berries (such as blueberries, raspberries, blackberries, etc.)

- 1 banana

- 1/2 cup plain yogurt

- 1/2 cup orange juice

- 2 tablespoons honey

Preparation:

- In a blender, combine the mixed berries, banana, yogurt, orange juice, and honey.

- Blend until smooth. Serve immediately.

7. Blueberry Oatmeal:

Ingredients:

- 1 cup rolled oats

- 1 cup milk

- 1/2 cup blueberries

- 1 tablespoon honey

- 1/2 teaspoon ground cinnamon

Preparation:

- In a saucepan, boil the milk. Add the oats and stir.

- Reduce heat to the low, and then simmer it for 5 minutes, stirring it occasionally.

- Remove from heat and stir in the blueberries, honey, and cinnamon.

- Serve warm.

8. Burritos Rapidos:

Ingredients:

- 4 burrito-size flour tortillas

- 1 cup cooked black beans

- 1 cup cooked rice

- 1/2 cup salsa

- 1/2 cup shredded cheese

- 1/4 cup chopped cilantro

- 1/4 cup diced red onion

- 1/4 cup diced bell pepper

- Salt and pepper to taste

Preparation:

- In a medium bowl, mix together the black beans, rice, salsa, cheese, cilantro, red onion, and bell pepper.

- Season it with salt and pepper.

- Place 1/4 of the filling in the center of each tortilla.

- Fold the sides of the tortilla over the filling, and then roll up the tortilla.

- Place the burritos on a baking sheet.

- Bake it in a preheated 350°F oven for like 15 minutes.

- Serve warm.

9. Fresh Fruit Lassi:

Ingredients:

- 1 cup plain yogurt

- 1/2 cup diced fresh fruit (such as mango, pineapple, strawberries, etc.)

- 1 tablespoon honey

- 1 teaspoon ground cardamom

- Ice cubes (optional)

Preparation:

- In a blender, combine the yogurt, diced fruit, honey, and cardamom.

- Blend until smooth.

- Add ice cubes (if using). Serve immediately.

10. Apple Filled Crepes:

Ingredients:

- 1 cup all-purpose flour

- 2 eggs

- 1 cup milk

- 2 tablespoons melted butter

- 2 tablespoons sugar

- 1/2 teaspoon ground cinnamon

- 2 apples, peeled, cored, and diced

- 2 tablespoons butter

- 2 tablespoons brown sugar

Preparation:

• In a medium bowl, whisk together the flour, eggs, milk, melted butter, sugar, and cinnamon.

• Heat a nonstick skillet over medium heat. Grease the skillet with a little butter.

• Pour 1/4 cup of the batter into the skillet and swirl to coat the bottom.

• Cook for 1 minute, or until golden brown. Flip and cook for 1 minute more.

• Transfer the crepe to a plate. Repeat with the remaining batter.

CHAPTER FOUR

Lunch Recipes for Kidney Transplant Diets

1. Apple Rice Salad

Ingredients:

- 2 cups cooked white rice

- 1/4 cup diced red onion

- 2 green onions, chopped

- 1/2 cup diced celery

- 2 large apples, cored and diced

- 1/2 cup dried cranberries

- 1/2 cup mayonnaise

- 2 tablespoons lemon juice

- Salt and pepper to taste

Preparation:

- In a large bowl, combine the cooked white rice, red onion, green onions, celery, apples, and dried cranberries.

- In another bowl, whisk together the mayonnaise, the lemon juice, salt, and pepper.

- Pour over the rice mixture and stir until everything is well blended.

- Serve cold or at room temperature.

2. Baked Potato Soup

Ingredients:

- 2 tablespoons butter

- 2 tablespoons all-purpose flour

- 2 cups chicken broth

- 2 cups milk

- 2 large baking potatoes, cooked it and cubed it

- 1/2 teaspoon salt

- 1/4 teaspoon black pepper

- 1/2 cup shredded cheddar cheese

- 2 tablespoons chopped fresh parsley

Preparation:

• In a bigger saucepan, melt the butter on average heat.

• Add the flour and stir it for 1 minute.

• Gradually add the chicken broth and the milk, stirring it constantly.

• Boil and reduce the heat then simmer it for like 5 minutes.

• Add the cubed potatoes, salt, and pepper, and simmer for an additional 10 minutes.

• Stir in the cheddar cheese and parsley just before serving.

3. Beef Barley Soup

Ingredients:

- 1 pound lean ground beef

- 1 tablespoon vegetable oil

- 1 onion, diced

- 2 carrots, diced

- 2 celery stalks, diced

- 2 garlic cloves, minced

- 6 cups beef broth

- 1 cup pearled barley

- 2 bay leaves

- 1 teaspoon dried thyme

- 1/2 teaspoon salt

- 1/4 teaspoon black pepper

Preparation:

- In a large pot, heat the vegetable oil on average-high heat.

- Add the ground beef, onion, carrots, celery, and garlic, and cook until the beef is browned.

- Add the beef broth, barley, bay leaves, thyme, salt, and pepper.

- Bring to a boil, then reduce heat and simmer for 45 minutes, stirring occasionally.

- Remove the bay leaves before serving.

4. Black Bean Burger

Ingredients:

- 1 (15-ounce) can black beans, drained it and rinsed it

- 1/2 cup breadcrumbs

- 1/2 cup diced onion

- 1/2 cup diced bell pepper

- 1/4 cup chopped fresh cilantro

- 1 teaspoon ground cumin

- 1 teaspoon garlic powder

- 1 teaspoon chili powder

- 2 tablespoons olive oil

- 4 hamburger buns

Preparation:

- In a bigger bowl, mash the black beans with fork.

- Add the breadcrumbs, onion, bell pepper, cilantro, cumin, garlic powder, and chili powder, and mix until everything is combined.

- Form the mixture into four patties.

- Heat the olive oil in a bigger skillet on average-high heat.

- Add the burgers and cook for 5 minutes per side, or until heated through.

- Serve on hamburger buns.

5. Chicken and Corn Chowder

Ingredients:

- 2 tablespoons butter

- 2 tablespoons all-purpose flour

- 2 cups chicken broth

- 2 cups milk

- 2 cups cooked, diced chicken

- 1 (15-ounce) can corn, drained

- 1/2 teaspoon salt

- 1/4 teaspoon black pepper

- 1/2 cup shredded cheddar cheese

- 2 tablespoons chopped fresh parsley

Preparation:

- In a bigger saucepan, melt the butter on average heat.

- Add the flour and stir it for 1 minute.

- Gradually add the chicken broth and the milk, stirring it constantly.

- Boil and reduce the heat then simmer it for like 5 minutes.

- Add the cooked chicken, corn, salt, and pepper, and simmer for an additional 10 minutes.

- Stir in the cheddar cheese and parsley just before serving.

6. Chicken and Dumplings

Ingredients:

- 2 tablespoons butter

- 2 tablespoons all-purpose flour

- 2 cups chicken broth

- 2 cups milk

- 2 cups cooked, diced chicken

- 2 cups biscuit mix

- 1/2 teaspoon salt

- 1/4 teaspoon black pepper

- 2 tablespoons chopped fresh parsley

Preparation:

- In a bigger saucepan, melt the butter on average heat.

- Add the flour and stir it for 1 minute.

- Gradually add the chicken broth and the milk, stirring it constantly.

- Boil and reduce the heat then simmer it for like 5 minutes.

- Add the cooked chicken, salt, and pepper, and simmer for an additional 10 minutes.

- In a separate bowl, mix the biscuit mix according to package instructions.

- Drop spoonfuls of biscuit dough into the simmering soup.

• Simmer it for an additional 10 minutes, or till the dumplings are cooked through. Stir in the parsley before serving.

7. Chicken N' Orange Salad Sandwich

Ingredients:

• 2 cups cooked, diced chicken

• 1/2 cup diced celery

• 1/2 cup diced red onion

• 1/2 cup diced green pepper

• 2 oranges, peeled and diced

• 1/2 cup mayonnaise

- 1/4 teaspoon salt

- 1/4 teaspoon black pepper

- 4 slices bread

Preparation:

- In a large bowl, combine the cooked chicken, celery, red onion, green pepper, and oranges.

- In a separate bowl, whisk together the mayonnaise, salt, and pepper.

- Pour over the chicken mixture and stir until everything is well blended.

- Spread the chicken salad onto the bread slices and serve.

8. Chinese Chicken Salad

Ingredients:

- 2 cups cooked, shredded chicken

- 1/2 cup diced celery

- 1/2 cup diced red onion

- 1/2 cup diced green pepper

- 2 tablespoons sesame oil

- 2 tablespoons soy sauce

- 1 tablespoon honey

- 1 teaspoon rice vinegar

- 2 tablespoons toasted sesame seeds

- 4 cups lettuce

Preparation:

- In a large bowl, combine the cooked chicken, celery, red onion, and green pepper.

- In a separate bowl, whisk together the sesame oil, soy sauce, honey, and rice vinegar.

- Pour over the chicken mixture and stir until everything is well blended.

- Sprinkle the toasted sesame seeds over the top.

- Serve over lettuce.

9. Cider Cream Chicken

Ingredients:

- 2 tablespoons butter

- 2 tablespoons all-purpose flour

- 2 cups chicken broth

- 2 cups milk

- 2 cups cooked, diced chicken

- 1/2 cup apple cider

- 1/4 cup heavy cream

- 1/2 teaspoon salt

- 1/4 teaspoon black pepper

- 2 tablespoons chopped fresh parsley

Preparation:

- In a bigger saucepan, melt the butter on average heat.

- Add the flour and stir it for 1 minute.

- Gradually add the chicken broth and the milk, stirring it constantly.

- Boil and reduce the heat then simmer it for like 5 minutes.

- Add the cooked chicken, apple cider, cream, salt, and pepper, and simmer for an additional 10 minutes.

- Stir in the parsley before serving.

10. Dijon Chicken Salad

Ingredients:

- 2 cups cooked, diced chicken

- 1/2 cup diced celery

- 1/2 cup diced red onion

- 1/2 cup diced green pepper

- 1/2 cup mayonnaise

- 2 tablespoons Dijon mustard

- 1 teaspoon honey

- 1/4 teaspoon salt

- 1/4 teaspoon black pepper

- 4 slices bread

Preparation:

● In a large bowl, combine the cooked chicken, celery, red onion, and green pepper.

● In another bowl, whisk together the mayonnaise, the Dijon mustard, the honey, salt, and pepper.

● Pour over the chicken mixture and stir until everything is well blended.

● Spread the chicken salad onto the bread slices and serve.

CHAPTER FIVE

Dinner Recipes for Kidney Transplant Diets

1. Confetti Chicken 'N Rice

Ingredients:

- 1 tablespoon vegetable oil

- 1 onion, chopped

- 1 green bell pepper, chopped

- 1½ cups long-grain white rice, uncooked

- 2 cloves garlic, minced

- 1 teaspoon chili powder

- 1 teaspoon ground cumin

- 2 cups chicken broth

- 1 (14.5-ounce) can diced tomatoes

- 1 (4-ounce) can diced green chilies

- 2 cups cooked, diced chicken

- ½ cup frozen corn

- ½ cup shredded cheese

Preparation:

- Heat oil in a bigger skillet on average-high heat.

- Add onion and the bell pepper and then cook till softened, for about 5 minutes.

- Add rice, garlic, chili powder, cumin, and oregano to the skillet and stir to combine.

- Pour in chicken broth, diced tomatoes, and green chilies. Stir to combine, reduce heat to low, and cover.

- Simmer it for like 20 minutes, till rice is cooked.

- Add chicken, corn, and cheese to the skillet.

- Stir to combine and cook until cheese is melted, about 5 minutes.

2. Crock Pot Chili Verde

Ingredients:

- 1 pound boneless pork, cut it into 1-inch cubes

- 1 (4-ounce) can diced green chilies

- 1 onion, chopped

- 2 cloves garlic, minced

- 1 (14.5-ounce) can diced tomatoes

- 1 cup chicken broth

- 2 tablespoons chili powder

- 1 teaspoon ground cumin

- 1 teaspoon dried oregano

- 1 (15-ounce) can white beans, drained it and rinsed it

Preparation:

• Place pork, green chilies, onion, garlic, diced tomatoes, chicken broth, chili powder, cumin, and oregano in a crock pot.

• Cover it and cook it on low for like 6-8 hours.

• Add beans and cook for an additional 30 minutes.

3.   Dilled Fish

Ingredients:

- 4 (6-ounce) salmon fillets

- 2 tablespoons olive oil

- Salt and pepper, to taste

- 2 tablespoons freshly chopped dill

- 2 tablespoons freshly squeezed lemon juice

Preparation:

- Preheat oven to 375°F.

- Place salmon fillets on a baking sheet lined with parchment paper.

- Drizzle with olive oil, season with salt and pepper, and sprinkle with dill.

- Bake for 15-20 minutes, until fish is cooked through.

- Drizzle with lemon juice before serving.

4. Easy Instant Pot Creamy Chicken Pasta

Ingredients:

- 2 tablespoons butter

- 1 onion, chopped

- 2 cloves garlic, minced

- 2 boneless, skinless chicken breasts, cut it into 1-inch cubes

- 1 (14.5-ounce) can diced tomatoes

- 1 cup chicken broth

- 1 teaspoon Italian seasoning

- 1 (8-ounce) package penne pasta

- 1 cup heavy cream

- 1 cup freshly grated Parmesan cheese

Preparation:

- Turn Instant Pot to sauté mode and add butter.

- Add the onion and the garlic and cook till softened, for about 5 minutes.

- Add chicken and cook until no longer pink, about 5 minutes.

- Add diced tomatoes, chicken broth, Italian seasoning, and pasta. Stir to combine.

- Lock the lid and set the pressure valve to sealing. Set to the manual high pressure for like 5 minutes.

- When the cooking time is complete, quick release the pressure.

- Stir in cream and Parmesan cheese.

- Serve and enjoy.

5. Fast Fajitas

Ingredients:

- 1 tablespoon vegetable oil

- 1 onion, sliced

- 1 red bell pepper, sliced

- 1 green bell pepper, sliced

- 2 cloves garlic, minced

- 1 teaspoon chili powder

- 1 teaspoon ground cumin

- 1 teaspoon dried oregano

- 1 pound boneless, skinless chicken breasts, cut it into 1-inch cubes

- Salt and pepper, to taste

- Flour or corn tortillas, for serving

Preparation:

• Heat oil in a large skillet over medium-high heat. Add onion and bell peppers and cook until softened, about 5 minutes.

• Add garlic, chili powder, cumin, and oregano to the skillet and stir to combine.

• Add chicken to the skillet and season with salt and pepper. Cook it till chicken is cooked through, for about 10 minutes.

• Serve chicken mixture in tortillas and enjoy.

6. Fast Roast Chicken with Lemon & Herbs

Ingredients:

- 1 tablespoon olive oil

- 1 whole chicken, cut into 8 pieces

- 1 lemon, cut into wedges

- 1 tablespoon freshly chopped rosemary

- 1 tablespoon freshly chopped thyme

- Salt and pepper, to taste

Preparation:

- Preheat oven to 375°F.

- Place chicken on a baking sheet lined with parchment paper.

- Drizzle with olive oil and top with lemon wedges.

- Sprinkle with rosemary and thyme and season with salt and pepper.

- Bake it for like 30-35 minutes, till chicken is cooked through.

7. Fresh Marinara Sauce

Ingredients:

- 2 tablespoons olive oil

- 1 onion, chopped

- 2 cloves garlic, minced

- 1 (28-ounce) can crushed tomatoes

- 1 (14.5-ounce) can diced tomatoes

- 2 tablespoons freshly chopped basil

- 2 tablespoons freshly chopped oregano

- Salt and pepper, to taste

Preparation:

- Heat olive oil in a bigger saucepan on average heat. Add onion and garlic and cook until softened, about 5 minutes.

- Add crushed tomatoes, diced tomatoes, basil, and oregano. Simmer for 30 minutes.

- Season with salt and pepper, to taste.

8. Fruit Vinegar Chicken

Ingredients:

- 2 tablespoons olive oil

- 4 boneless, skinless chicken breasts

- 1 onion, chopped

- 1 red bell pepper, chopped

- 1 cup apple cider vinegar

- 1 cup orange juice

- 1 teaspoon dried oregano

- Salt and pepper, to taste

Preparation:

• Heat olive oil in a bigger skillet on average-high heat. Add chicken and then cook till golden brown, for about like 5 minutes per side.

• Add onion and bell pepper and cook until softened, about 5 minutes.

• Reduce heat to low and add apple cider vinegar, orange juice, and oregano. Simmer it till chicken is cooked through, for about 10 minutes.

• Season it with salt and with pepper, to taste.

9. Fruity Chicken Salad

Ingredients:

- 2 tablespoons olive oil

- 4 boneless, skinless chicken breasts

- Salt and pepper, to taste

- 2 cups mixed greens

- 1 cup diced fresh fruit (such as apples, pears, grapes, or mangoes)

- ½ cup shredded cheese

- ¼ cup toasted pecans

- ¼ cup honey mustard dressing

Preparation:

• Heat olive oil in a bigger skillet on average-high heat.

• Add chicken and then cook till golden brown, for about like 5 minutes per side.

• Season it with salt and with pepper.

• In a large bowl, combine greens, fresh fruit, cheese, and pecans.

• Slice cooked chicken and add to salad.

• Drizzle it with honey mustard dressing and toss it to combine.

10. Grilled Salmon with Fruit Salsa

Ingredients:

- 4 (6-ounce) salmon fillets

- 2 tablespoons olive oil

- Salt and pepper, to taste

- 1 cup diced fresh fruit (such as apples, pears, grapes, or mangoes)

- 2 tablespoons freshly chopped cilantro

- 2 tablespoons freshly squeezed lime juice

Preparation:

- Preheat grill to medium-high heat.

- Place salmon fillets on a greased grill grate.

- Drizzle it with olive oil and then season it with salt and pepper.

- Grill for 6-8 minutes per side, until fish is cooked through.

- Meanwhile, in a medium bowl, combine diced fruit, cilantro, and lime juice.

- Serve salmon topped with fruit salsa and enjoy.

CHAPTER Six

Desserts Recipes for Kidney Transplant Diets

1. Asian Pear Torte

Ingredients:

- 3 Asian pears, peeled, cored and sliced it

- 2/3 cup all-purpose flour

- 1/2 cup butter, melted

- 1/2 cup white sugar

- 1/4 teaspoon ground cinnamon

- 1/4 teaspoon ground nutmeg

- 1/4 teaspoon ground cardamom

- 1/2 teaspoon vanilla extract

Preparation:

- Preheat oven to 350 degrees F.

- Grease a 9 inch round cake pan. Mix together flour, melted butter, sugar, cinnamon, nutmeg, and cardamom until crumbly.

- Place half of the mixture into the prepared pan.

- Arrange pear slices on top of mixture in pan.

- Sprinkle the remaining crumb mixture over the pears.

- Bake in preheated oven for 30 minutes.
- Allow to cool before serving.

2. Blueberry Whipped Pie

Ingredients:

- 1 (9 inch) prepared graham cracker crust

- 1 (8 oz) package cream cheese, softened

- 1/4 cup white sugar

- 1/4 teaspoon ground cinnamon

- 1 teaspoon vanilla extract

- 1 (8 oz) container frozen whipped topping, thawed it

- 2 cups fresh blueberries

Preparation:

- In a bowl, mix together the cream cheese, the sugar, the cinnamon and the vanilla until smooth.

- Fold in whipped topping until well blended.

- Spoon mixture into prepared crust.

- Top with blueberries. Refrigerate till chilled, at least for 2 hours.

3. Caramel Custard

Ingredients:

- 1/2 cup white sugar

- 2 tablespoons water

- 2 cups whole milk

- 1/3 cup white sugar

- 3 eggs

- 1 teaspoon vanilla extract

Preparation:

- Preheat oven to 350 degrees F.

- In a small saucepan, melt 1/2 cup sugar and water together over medium heat.

- Cook until the sugar is melted and the mixture is a light golden brown.

- Pour the caramel in a 9 inch round cake pan.

- In a medium bowl, mix together the milk, 1/3 cup sugar, eggs, and vanilla extract. Pour the mixture on the caramel in the cake pan.

- Place the pan in a bigger baking dish. Pour enough hot water into the larger dish to come halfway up the sides of the cake pan.

- Bake for 40 to 45 minutes in the preheated oven, or until set. Allow to cool before serving.

4. Carrot Muffins

Ingredients:

- 2 cups all-purpose flour

- 1/2 cup white sugar

- 2 teaspoons baking powder

- 1/2 teaspoon baking soda

- 1/2 teaspoon ground cinnamon

- 1/4 teaspoon ground nutmeg

- 1/4 teaspoon salt

- 2 eggs

- 1/2 cup vegetable oil

- 1/4 cup milk

- 1 teaspoon vanilla extract

- 1 1/2 cups grated carrots

Preparation:

- Preheat oven to 375 degrees F.

- Grease 12 muffin cups or line it with paper muffin liners.

- In a bigger bowl, mix together the flour, the sugar, the baking powder, the baking soda, cinnamon, nutmeg and salt.

- In a another bowl, whisk together the eggs, oil, milk and the vanilla.

- Stir the wet ingredients with the dry ingredients till combined. Fold in the grated carrots.

- Divide the batter to the prepared muffin cups.

- Bake in preheated oven for 18 to 20 minutes, or until a toothpick inserted into a muffin comes out clean.

5. Cheesecake

Ingredients:

- 1 1/2 cups graham cracker crumbs

- 2 tablespoons white sugar

- 1/3 cup butter, melted

- 3 (8 oz) packages cream cheese, softened

- 1 cup white sugar

- 3 eggs

- 1 teaspoon vanilla extract

- 1/4 cup all-purpose flour

- 1/2 cup sour cream

Preparation:

- Preheat oven to 325 degrees F.

- Grease a 9 inch springform pan.

- In a bowl, mix together the graham cracker crumbs, 2 tablespoons sugar, and the melted butter.

- Press it into the bottom and up the sides of the prepared pan.

• Bake in preheated oven for 8 minutes. In a large bowl, beat cream cheese and 1 cup sugar until smooth.

• Beat in eggs, one at a time, mixing just until blended. Blend in vanilla, flour, and sour cream.

• Pour filling into prepared crust. Bake in preheated oven for 40 minutes. Allow to cool before serving.

CHAPTER Seven

Snacks Recipes for Kidney Transplant Diets

1. Beef Jerky

Ingredients:

- 2 pounds lean beef, sliced into thin strips

- 1/4 cup soy sauce

- 2 tablespoons Worcestershire sauce

- 1 teaspoon garlic powder

- 1 teaspoon onion powder

- 1/4 teaspoon ground black pepper

Preparation:

- Preheat oven to 200 degrees F.

- Line a baking sheet with aluminum foil.

- In a medium bowl, mix together soy sauce, Worcestershire sauce, garlic powder, onion powder, and pepper.

- Place the beef strips in the marinade and mix to coat.

- Arrange the beef strips on prepared baking sheet.

- Bake 4 to 5 hours in the preheated oven, or until beef is dry and leathery.

2. Brown Bag Popcorn

Ingredients:

- 1/4 cup popcorn kernels

- 1 brown paper lunch bag

- 1 teaspoon vegetable oil

- Salt to taste

Preparation:

- Pour the popcorn kernels and vegetable oil into the brown paper bag.

- Fold the top of the bag over twice, and staple it shut.

- Place the bag in the microwave and cook on high for 2 to 3 minutes, or until popping slows.

- Carefully remove the bag from the microwave and season with salt to taste.

3. Cornbread Muffins

Ingredients:

- 1 cup cornmeal

- 1 cup all-purpose flour

- 1/4 cup white sugar

- 1 teaspoon baking powder

- 1/2 teaspoon baking soda

- 1/2 teaspoon salt

- 1 egg

- 1 cup buttermilk

- 1/4 cup vegetable oil

Preparation:

- Preheat oven to 400 degrees F.

- Grease 12 muffin cups or line it with paper muffin liners.

- In a bigger bowl, mix together the cornmeal, flour, sugar, baking powder, baking soda, and salt.

- In another bowl, whisk together the egg, the buttermilk, and oil. Stir the wet ingredients with the dry ingredients just until blended.

- Divide the batter to the prepared muffin cups.

- Bake in preheated oven for 18 to 20 minutes, or until a toothpick inserted into a muffin comes out clean.

4. Ginger Cranberry Punch

Ingredients:

- 4 cups cranberry juice

- 4 cups pineapple juice

- 1 (2 liter) bottle ginger ale

- 2 cups orange juice

- 2 cups frozen cranberries

- 2 tablespoons fresh grated ginger

- 1 lime, sliced

Preparation:

- In a large punch bowl or pitcher, mix together cranberry juice, pineapple juice, ginger ale, orange juice, frozen cranberries, grated ginger, and lime slices.

- Serve chilled.

5. Joyce's Quick Dip

Ingredients:

- 1 (8 oz) package cream cheese, softened

- 1 (8 oz) container sour cream

- 1 (1 oz) package dry Italian-style salad dressing mix

- 1/4 cup sliced green onions

- 1/2 cup chopped fresh mushrooms

- 1/2 cup chopped bell pepper

Preparation:

• In a medium bowl, mix together cream cheese, sour cream, salad dressing mix, green onions, mushrooms, and bell pepper.

• Chill it for at least 2 hours before serving.

• Serve with crackers or chips.

Conclusion

This cookbook is an invaluable resource that provides a wide range of recipes tailored to the needs of those who have had or are about to undergo a kidney transplant.

The recipes are easy to follow, nutritionally balanced, and appealing to the taste buds.

Whether you are a patient, caregiver, or healthcare practitioner, this cookbook is a great resource for providing a nutritionally balanced diet for pre and post-transplant patients.

Made in the USA
Las Vegas, NV
11 December 2023

82505292R00079